Reset Your Life in 30 Days

Reset Your Life in 30 Days

A Guide to Detox Your Mind, Body & Spirit

ALLISON LIDDLE

ALLISON LIDDLE CONSULTING, LLC
WAUSAU, WI

Copyright 2021. All Rights Reserved. This book or any portion thereof may not be reproduced or used in any manner whatsoever without the express written permission of the author, except for the use of brief quotations in a book review or journal. Library of Congress Control Number: 2021904216

Dedication

I dedicate this book to my amazing sister, Anika.

I am so proud of you every day.

Keep on being you.

The world needs your brilliant light.

Love you!

Sissy

Contents

Introduction	1
	5
Day 1: More Reflection, Less Social Media	7
Day 2: More Positivity, Less Negativity	11
Day 3: More Healthy Food, Less Sugar/Processed Food	15
Day 4: More Gratitude, Less Complaining	19
Day 5: More Healthy Habits, Less Unhealthy Habits	22
Day 6: More Meditation, Less Chaos	25
Day 7: More Lifters, Less Drainers	27
Day 8: More Planning, Less Overwhelm	29
Day 9: More Love, Less Stress	33
Day 10: More Water, Less Unhealthy Drinks	36
Day 11: More Joy, Less Sadness	38
Day 12: More Happiness, Less Unhappiness	40
Day 13: More Relaxation, Less Worry	43
Day 14: More Healing, Less Pain	46
Day 15: More Acceptance, Less Judgment	49
Day 16: More Togetherness, Less Separation	52
Day 17: More Reading, Less Screen/Computer Time	55
Day 18: More Nature Time, Less Indoor Time	58
Day 19: More Intentionality, Less Hustle	61

Day 20: More Slow, Less Hurry	64
Day 21: More Responsibility, Less Blaming Questions	67
Day 22: Which activity was your favorite? Why?	69
Day 23: How are you feeling?	71
Day 24: What's one fun thing you could do today? Do it!	73
Day 25: Celebrate your accomplishments, write them down.	75
Day 26: Create a list of 10 positive words to describe yourself. Read them out loud daily.	77
Day 27: Thank yourself for being committed to growth.	80
Day 28: More Abundance, Less Scarcity	82
Day 29: Pay it forward!	85
Day 30: Review of Your Reset	87
Thank You	90
About the Author	92
NOTES:	96

Introduction

Have you ever been in the cycle of stress and fear wondering what you should add to your plate to make it "simpler." Me too, and I realized adding doesn't work.

On September 15, 2019, I received a message from the universe to reset my life. The message told me to focus more on being and less on doing. So, I listened... the first time.

I say I listened the first time because there have been many, many, many times when I received a message and rather than listening and surrendering to it, I said, "Really? You want me to do that? It doesn't make sense. It won't work for me. Maybe later." However, this year I've continually had the message to surrender; finally, after years of not listening, I just did it.

I want to give you a picture of my life when I received this message. I was overworked, stressed to the maximum (adrenal fatigue, which meant my body couldn't handle the stress anymore), overwhelmed, frustrated, and exhausted. I was struggling to keep it going and the last thing I thought I needed to do was to stop and reset my life. My solution was to add yet another thing to my plate. I'll do more yoga... I'll meditate for an hour a day... I'll build my business bigger... I'll work out harder... I'll hustle... I'll find a coach... I'll write a book... I'll create a new product... I'll revamp my brand.

Here's the huge problem in our society right now. We feel like the solution to whatever problem we are facing is found by adding more to our lives, not stopping things. We've been conditioned to believe if we just buy the book, join the course, take the class, buy the outfit, go on the vacation, or work harder then we'll meet the solution we seek of taming the chaos of our lives. Unfortunately, life doesn't work like this. Adding more will not create clarity. Doing more will not calm you down. Hustling will not build your business. Making yourself absolutely miserable will not make your life happier.

As I write it, my guess is you're nodding your head because I was thinking to myself, Well, of course, those things won't help create a calm, happy, fulfilled life. However, we live in the information age and we're bombarded with more information than ever before in history. Access to information isn't the problem, I think the real problem is the fact that we now can compare our lives to the lives of others in real-time all day, every day. All of the comparing and judging leads to frustration, stress, and worry. Too much of our time is spent in the world of the fake lives of others and we wonder why they can do so much, have so much time, or are so accomplished. The reality of social media is even the "real" people are not sharing the whole story because they typically can't online.

I'm very aware of the compare game and the negative affects it can have on confidence, but even I was feeling the pressure to keep up and do more. The funny thing is I was trying to keep up and do more to an unrealistic version of "success." Have you ever done that?

This guide was written for the person who is struggling with life and wondering what the heck else you can do. Your plate is overflowing so much that if you add even one more crumb to it, it'll shatter into a million pieces. You feel like you're walking through your life in a fog of stress, plagued by constant guilt of not being able to please everyone. You've neglected your own self-care because really who has the time for that stuff, right? You've pretty much given in to the fact your life will just continue to feel this miserable... or if not miserable, difficult. You spend your days fantasizing about your next vacation because then you'll at least have a week off from worrying about the reality of your life.

My dear friend, if you can relate to any of what I just said, I'm giving you're a virtual hug. I've been there and I know how it feels. On September 15, I too felt that exact same way and I had no clue what to do next. I think the message God gave me is for you too. I truly believe in order to really understand another person you must first have experienced some of the pain they have felt. In that pain, you're able to understand your own struggle, and when you overcome it, you're able to emerge stronger, more confident, and ready to help others.

Reset Your Life in 30 Days will help you go from chaos to clarity in your life. You'll learn practical tools to help you stop, reflect, and let go of the parts of life holding you back from designing a life you love.

The book will outline 30 simple ways to detox your mind, body, and spirit in 30 days. (If you miss a day, or a week, just start up again.) You can use this book in many different ways. You could read it and go through all of the exercises in order. Perhaps you use the book depending on the struggle you are facing in your life right now. All I can say is I recommend you go through the whole book for 30 days straight. There is something magical about committing to yourself to reset your life. You'll gain confidence in knowing you stuck to it. It reminds me of the time when my husband gave up Starbucks coffee for a whole year. The number one thing he learned was his own power to commit and take action in his life. It's led to him growing in all areas of his life. Don't underestimate the power of the simplicity of these principles. When applied, they can literally reset your life.

QUESTION: But really, Allison, why should I spend 30 days to reset your life?

Yesterday my father passed away.

I know that's a bold way to explain why you need to stop to reset your life, but it's true.

You see, my father and I were not close. There was a long history of addiction and disease in his life, and as an adult, I finally decided to create boundaries to protect myself and my family from the pain.

Thirty days ago, I reset my life without knowing exactly why, but I now know why I needed to do that reset. I now understand that it was necessary in order to deal with this difficult situation with clarity and power.

Have you ever gotten one of those whispers and listened to it? Not exactly understanding why, but just feeling in your soul that you needed to listen? Well, that is what happened to me 30 days ago, and to be honest I didn't want to reset my life. I didn't think I needed a reset in my life. I had too much to do, be, and have. I had goals, people. Big, huge, audacious goals, and what would happen to those goals if I just let them be?

If you are a high achiever like me, the thought of stopping or even slowing down what you are doing may cause you stress. I get it. I was absolutely there. I did not in any way want to lose my momentum. I love working. I love achieving goals. I love helping people. I love all of it.

Today, one day after the passing of my father I recognize the power of the reset. I would not have been able to deal with this obstacle with grace if I had not slowed down. I'm 99% sure I would have probably lost my mind a bit, and not only that, I would not be able to handle the stress of this difficult situation without falling into stress coping mechanisms.

And on top of all that, death has a way of helping me put life into perspective. The things I thought were so stressful suddenly don't really seem like a big deal. The little things I had been taking for granted now seem like the most important things to me. This shift in perspective helped me fully appreciate the power of the RESET. Even in the struggle of life right now, the lessons I'm learning are putting me here to hopefully serve you so you can take the time to move intentionally into your life today and not wait until it's too late.

I share all of this to tell you that right now, as you read this guide, you may not have clarity into the future. My sincere hope is that your reset is for some amazing opportunity brewing. Are you ready to detox your mind, body, and spirit? YAY! I'm so excited for you.

Day 1: More Reflection, Less Social Media

"Where your focus goes your energy flows." – Emerson

The day I gave up social media for 30 days I felt like I couldn't possibly do it. I'd been waking up each day with social media, checking it throughout the day, and checking it one last time before bed each day. It was an all-consuming obsession in my life and I justified the amount of time with the idea that I was "building my tribe" or "building my brand." (FYI: This is complete crap I fed myself to justify this distraction.)

Someone is reading this and saying, "Yes, me too. I'm building and I need to engage. My business won't grow if I'm not on social media." And perhaps all of your business is on social media, I dunno. I just know that I thought a similar thing. I thought if I don't hop on to answer, like, share, etc., then I won't be able to grow my business. However, after going through the 30-day challenge, I learned that it was a false belief.

Do you take time each day to reflect on your actions? Imagine having the time and freedom to reflect on your actions and be able to clearly understand what your next step is.

In the introduction, I talk about where I was at in my health when I started the 30-day challenge. I was stressed out, overwhelmed, and struggling to "hustle." (Can we throw out this dang word? I really have come to despise it because I know we're all doing more than people did 20-30 years ago, and yet we're dealing with more mental health issues, more people struggling, and less connection in our families.)

So, there I was, wondering what the heck was wrong with me. I thought that perhaps I needed to go on a retreat weekend to "reset." Or maybe see a therapist. Perhaps there would be a book at Barnes

& Noble that would help me figure out why I was struggling to keep going at that insane pace of life.

In walks the "Reset Your Life in 30 Days" idea.

To be completely honest with you, I thought there was no way cutting things out of my life was going to help me. I thought this was absolutely not the solution. Maybe it was the solution for other people, but it would not work for me. It's too simple. It's too easy.

Cut out some stuff like social media, add in some good things like meditation, yoga, and exercise, and in 30 days, I'd feel better. I didn't think it could be that simple, but it actually was, and in this guide, I'm going to walk you through the process.

Day 1: More Reflection, Less Social Media Questions

What is the date today?

———————————————————————————

What is the date in 30 days?

———————————————————————————

Now put the end of your 30 day reset into your calendar.

———————————————————————————

What social media are you currently on?

———————————————————————————

———————————————————————————

How much time do you think you are taking on social media daily?

_____

Now I want you to delete all social media apps from your phone and log out of your accounts on your computer. This is real, friend and you can do it.

_____

Right now how would you rate your current stress/ overwhelm level 1-10 (10 being really stinkin' stressed out)

_____

In 30 days if this crazy idea worked and you reset your life how would it feel to you?

_____
_____

If you were going to describe the emotions you feel most during the day what would you say they are?

_____
_____
_____
_____

Looking at those emotions, do you feel like they are serving the best version of you? Why or why not?

_____

_____

_____

_____

Day 2: More Positivity, Less Negativity

"Be positive. Your mind is more powerful than you think. What is down in the well comes up in the bucket. Fill yourself with positive things." – Tony Dungy

Today we're going to help you do something to literally shift your life forever. Am I exaggerating? Nope.

One of the things I pride myself on is being one of the most enthusiastic and positive people I know. In college, I had a boss who smile-talked. Have you ever met one of those people? It's funny. Anywho, the smile-talker was positive all of the time. He was also very successful in his chosen career. I was fascinated with his ability to see the good in every situation, even the really difficult ones. I'd never met anyone who looked at the bright side of absolutely everything. I remember one day I was going into the football locker room to put away their laundry. Did I mention I washed laundry for the athletic department? It was gross and fun at the same time. I wore really big gloves so it felt like I was a scientist or something. (I sound a bit crazy, I know, but I needed a job to pay for college and it allowed me to do homework while the laundry washed.)

While I was putting away the laundry, singing to myself, I decided I would start to intentionally be more positive. I started with my thoughts. I decided I would start being intentional about being more positive in my mind. Each day I would examine my thoughts: were they positive or negative? When did I feel the best or the worst? I have always had a serious case of getting "hangry," so when I'm hungry or tired my, thoughts and attitude would be more negative. In the morning, after a cup of coffee, I would feel energized and happy. By mid-morning, when I was in a quiet room and focused on my work, I could get so much done and I was in a positive frame of mind. After lunch I was sleepy, so I'd typically take a short 20-minute nap, and then I'd be recharged. I continued to monitor my thoughts hour by hour throughout the day. In this analysis, I found some key ideas.

1. There were specific times during the day when I was more positive naturally.
2. If I was hungry or tired, I needed to take a break.
3. I needed to recharge myself through a nap or exercise.
4. I could observe my thoughts and evaluate whether they were positive or negative.
5. I could choose what thoughts I wanted to keep, so I chose the positive ones.

Choose positive thoughts, evaluate your daily patterns, and use this research to help set yourself up for success.

In the first sentence of this day, I said this one section could transform your life, and I said that to you because I believe it can. I believe you have the power, through your thoughts to design a life you absolutely love. The opposite is also true. If you decide to choose destructive thoughts, you could ruin your life. Choose wisely.

Day 2: More Positivity, Less Negativity Questions:

Would you describe yourself as more positive or negative?

_____

_____

What's your favorite time of day? Do you feel happy, focused, and energized at this time? (i.e., morning, afternoon, evening, late night)

_____

_____

Do you find your emotions are more negative if you are hungry, stressed, or tired?

_____

_____

Did you know we cycle through about 8-10 emotions in a given week? What emotions do you feel most often?

_____

_____

Review the emotions you wrote down. Are they positive or negative?

_____

_____

If you envision your best self, what emotions dominate your life in your best version?

_____

_____

What actions can you take to be happier? (i.e., sing, listen to music, work out, laugh, talk to a loved one, etc.)

_____

_____

If you could create a daily routine to help you be more positive what would it be?

_____

_____

Who are the most positive influences in your life? What do they do specifically to be positive?

_____

_____

Reflecting on your answers from today, what is the one thing you could start doing to become more positive?

_____

_____

Day 3: More Healthy Food, Less Sugar/Processed Food

"Take care of your health first because a healthy body can take care of everything." Megha

You get one body for your entire life. That's it. I find too often that people do not understand this fact of life until it's too late.

After my daughter Avery was born, I decided to start leading a healthier lifestyle because I wanted to be around for my children until I was 150 years old. I figured I better start eating healthier and exercising if I wanted that goal to happen.

What's healthy food?

Here's the deal. I didn't really understand what "healthy" food was when I started my health journey. I'd heard of people only drinking shakes, eating veggies, or taking diet pills, but I wanted to learn how to eat healthy forever, so the short-term fix wasn't what I needed.

After some research, I found an app called Fooducate that would help me understand labels and rank the food for how healthy it was. It worked and now I know how to read food labels, and I try to eat whole foods. I also drink a lot of water and have replaced my sugary/diet sodas with ice tea or water. I try to get at least half my body weight in ounces every day. In my research I found that many of my problems were coming from not drinking enough water. Did you know if you're dehydrated you'll feel hungry? Or if you're tired, it could be because you need to drink water? Water is so good for you.

What if I hate to exercise?

I hated to exercise. I really did not like it, and to make it worse, I'd remind myself how hard it was and how much I hated it the entire time I worked out. The thing that worked for me was to switch my belief about exercise. It took practice, but I replaced my belief that "I hate exercise" to "I love how I feel after I exercise. I feel strong, and it clears my head."

After a few weeks of replacing this belief, I started to actually like exercise and I would make time in my schedule to get my workout in. What I realized is that in order to be the healthiest version of ourselves, the first thing we need to do is just to start. Move your body, take a walk, just do something to sweat. Then, eventually, you'll want to move your body and stay healthy.

These are my two life hacks for staying healthy: eating right by learning how to read labels and exercising. I know this isn't too complicated, but when you apply it for some time, my guess is that you'll feel healthier, look healthier, and have more energy.

Here's to a healthier you!

Day 3: More Healthy Food, Less Sugar/Processed Food Questions:

Would you describe yourself as healthy or unhealthy in your eating?

_____

_____

_____

If you were going to change one thing about your current health routine what would it be?

_____

_____

Do you move your body regularly to break a sweat?

_____

_____

What is one way you could start moving your body today? (i.e., go for a walk, run, bike, hike, swim, dance)

_____

_____

Start to track your eating habits today in a notebook for the next month with the calories. Are most of the food fresh or processed? Do you eat at restaurants often?

_____

_____

If you could create a daily routine to help you be more healthy in your eating what would you do?

_____

_____

Who are the healthiest people in your life? Or where could you find them?

_____

_____

Reflecting on your answers from today, what is the one thing you could start doing to become more healthy?

_____

_____

Day 4: More Gratitude, Less Complaining

Definition of Gratitude: the quality of being thankful; readiness to show appreciation for and to return kindness

I'm a pretty optimistic person. Every day I wake up and think to myself, *Another great day in paradise, let's do this!*

I understand that not everybody wakes up like this, and I didn't wake up like this for many years. Then I started to practice gratitude daily and it completely changed my attitude toward life.

Trust me, there are still those days when I get frustrated or overwhelmed. I actually am having days where I'm pushed to make more decisions and bigger decisions that will impact many more people than ever before. I don't take the responsibility I have lightly, so yes, there can be tough days.

But I've found some life-changing practices that turn bad days into awesome, amazing, wonderful, spectacular, pinch-me, happiness days. For real!

1) **Be Intentional**: Look for the good in every single situation, good or bad. If it's a tough situation you can say out loud, "What lesson am I learning right now?" Then write it down or teach it as soon as you can, so if someone else is going through a similar situation, they can learn the lesson too.

2) **Practice Gratitude**: You can do this in various ways. You can write down what you're grateful for, but what I enjoy even more is the act of showing gratitude by writing a thank you, sending a text to a friend, surprising my family with a gift, paying for a stranger's coffee at the coffee shop, or giving away a book. Something that is an action to express gratitude switches a bad day into an awesome day.

3) **Be Thankful to Be Alive**: Are you thankful you're alive? I've had two near-death experiences and three cancer scares. When I think a day is really bad, I remind myself about how it's probably not that bad. I'm alive, I have a beautiful family, wonderful friends, amazing opportunities to serve people I absolutely love. How could I see bad in that?

I hope this helps you change your perspective from a bad day into an awesome, amazing, wonderful, spectacular, pinch-me, happiness day.

Day 4: More Gratitude, Less Complaining Questions:

Do you regularly practice gratitude?

_____

_____

_____

Make a list of everything in your life to be grateful for today.

_____

_____

_____

_____

Sometimes we fall into patterns of complaining. What do you think you complain about the most?

What is one way you could start practicing gratitude daily?

Who are the most grateful people in your life?

Reflecting on your answers from today, what is the one thing you could start doing to focus on gratitude more often?

Day 5: More Healthy Habits, Less Unhealthy Habits

"The first wealth is health" – Ralph Waldo Emerson

How many of us know that we should change some of our health habits, but feel overwhelmed by where to start? Me too!

Let's make this easy and fun. If things are easy and fun, it's much more likely that we'll stick to them and we'll achieve the goal we set out to achieve.

FIVE TO LAUNCH:

1. Get an extra hour of sleep. Research shows we need more sleep, not less. Set your bedtime one hour earlier to get into bed. Aim for 7-9 hours of uninterrupted sleep each night.

2. Move your body for 30 minutes daily. Get in the habit of moving your body every single day. Aim for 30 minutes of exercising in some way.

3. Drink more water. Did you know 60% of our body is made up of water? Drink half of your body weight in water each day. Yes, really. Go buy yourself a big water bottle and drink water all day long. Yes, you'll make more visits to the restroom, but it'll help your body operate more effectively and you'll feel more energized.

4. Choose fresh foods. Fresh fruits and vegetables are an important part of a healthy diet. They contain essential vitamins, minerals, fiber, and other nutrients that are essential for good health.

5. Practice being happy. Being more positive and grateful can impact every area of your life. Your mindset will influence every single area of your life. Grab a journal and start writing down what you are grateful for every day and what you are looking forward to. Be happy. Have fun. Laugh and enjoy life. It'll make a difference.

Day 5: More Healthy Habits, Less Unhealthy Habits Questions:

START FIVE TO LAUNCH:

Get an extra hour of sleep. Research shows we need more sleep, not less. Set your bedtime one hour earlier to get into bed. 7-9 hours is ideal.

*How many hours of uninterrupted sleep am I getting each night? How could I increase this? *Note: if you are not getting that many hours, go in to see a medical professional.*

_____

_____

_____

Move your body for 30 minutes daily. Get in the habit of moving your body every single day for 30 minutes through exercise (ideas: walking, running, biking, hiking, swimming, dancing, strength training, etc).

Do I currently move my body 30 minutes daily? If not, what could I start doing?

_____

_____

_____

Drink more water. Did you know 60% of our body is made up of water?

How many ounces of water do I need to drink to reach my goal of ½ my body weight in ounces?

_____

_____

_____

Choose fresh foods. Fresh fruits and vegetables are an important part of a healthy diet. They contain essential vitamins, minerals, fiber, and other nutrients that are essential for good health. How many servings of fruits and veggies do you currently eat daily?

_____

_____

_____

Practice being happy. Being more positive and grateful can impact every area of your life. How often am I happy? Why?

_____

_____

_____

Day 6: More Meditation, Less Chaos

"Your goal is not to battle with the mind, but to witness the mind." – Swami Muktananda

Have you ever heard the word "meditation"? If I say that word to my husband, he calls me a "hippie." Haha! In all seriousness, this one word could be the ultimate gift you learn during this reset process. Meditation is the practice of clearing out your mind and focusing on your breath. When I was 16 years old, I suffered from anxiety. I was worried about everything from my grades, to my hair, if those people liked me, and if I'd get into college. Then I'd be worried about being worried. If you've ever lived with anxiety, you probably know what I'm talking about. It's not fun at all and it can consume you if you allow it to. If you are suffering from mental health issues, I always recommend you seek out professional help first. I did that too and it's okay to ask for help. In my case, I was letting the chaos of life consume me, which led to me feeling worried.

But then, one of my friends suggested I attend a yoga class. I remember the first class felt awkward. I didn't understand the breathing and movement. I couldn't do most of the moves, but then, at the end of class, the teacher told us to lie on our mats and breathe. I could do this! I laid down. Again, the anxiety rushed into my brain, but slowly, as I breathed deeper, I felt the tension leave my body. My thoughts slowed down and I felt so much better.

Meditation works to help you get control of your brain and body connection. You become an observer of your thoughts. After some practice, you may even realize when you need to meditate to slow your thinking down.

After 20 years of yoga and meditation, I'm hooked. In the action section, I'll walk you through a mediation process I use daily.

Day 6: More Mediation, Less Chaos Actions:

1. Find a quiet location to sit cross-legged on the floor.

2. Close your eyes.

3. For a count of 5, breathe in deeply filling your diaphragm.

4. For a count of 10, breathe out slowly.

5. Repeat this process while visualizing a special place you've been to (think island, beach, forest, etc.).

6. As your thoughts start to wander, bring them back into the present. Focus on your breathing. In for 5, out for 10, in for 5, out for 10.

7. After 3 minutes, open your eyes and notice how your body feels. It may feel tingly or light. Your mind may feel clearer.

8. Congratulate yourself for meditating. Take time each day to continue this practice.

Day 7: More Lifters, Less Drainers

"May your choices reflect your hopes, not your fears." – Nelson Mandela

I believe there is something good in every single person. However, when you are on a journey to become the best version of you, it helps to surround yourself with lifters. I'm going to help you understand what I mean.

A lifter is a person who is positive, encouraging, kind, friendly, caring, and wants the best for you. They see your strengths and remind you of them. These people are wonderful to have around you during your reset because they help you continue to focus on taking really good care of yourself. You are important. Every time you are around a lifter, you feel appreciated. Lifters are gifts.

A drainer is a negative person. This person may or may not be aware of their negative attitude. These people aren't just having a bad day or week; they are constantly negative in the way they talk, how they think, and the ways they behave. It is really difficult to be around drainers because it feels like all they can see is the bad things in the world. Many times after being around a drainer, you also will feel drained of energy.

In the reset, it is imperative for you to maintain your energy. In order to maintain your energy, you must guard it. One of the most effective ways to guard it is through evaluating who you are surrounding yourself with.

Choose wisely.

Day 7: More Lifters, Less Drainers

Why is positive, uplifting energy important to you and your success?

Who are some of the people in your life that encourage and lift you the most? Hint: These are your lifters.

Who are some of the people in your life that drain your energy? Hint: These are your drainers.

What do you need to do to spend more time with your lifters?

Day 8: More Planning, Less Overwhelm

"It takes as much energy to wish as it does to plan." – Eleanor Roosevelt

I'm a mom, wife, business owner (two businesses), sister, daughter, friend, author, and the list goes on.

I'll be perfectly honest. For a long time, I did not intentionally think about planning out my life or time. I ran around feeling overwhelmed most of the time, forgetting important things, and wondering why it felt like everyone else had it so "together."

Then one of my mentors said, "Allison, you have the same amount of time as everyone else. How you use your time matters."

Think about it. You are gifted 24 hours a day, about 30 days a month, and 365 days a year. How you and I choose to spend our time matters.

The first thing I did is track how much time I was spending doing everything in my life for a whole week. I created lists for each area of my life: home, work, fitness, family, faith, fun.

After a week of tracking my time, I reviewed where I was spending the most time. I quickly realized there were items I could eliminate right away because I knew they were not serving the best version of me. TV was one of those items. I turned off the TV and got back five hours! WOW, this stuff works.

Next was choosing the items I needed to consistently do in order to become the best version of me. I picked five areas: faith time, family time, fitness time, finances/field, fun. In my planner, I started to schedule out my entire week making sure I had time allotted for each of these areas.

Then I transferred all of the items I had just scheduled and put them into my online calendar.

The first time I did this it felt awkward, but soon I was a planning machine. After planning like this for a few weeks, I recognized that my overwhelm dissipated because I felt more in control of my time.

Day 8: More Planning, Less Overwhelm Questions:

This week track where you are spending your time.

Monday	Tuesday	Wednesday	Thursday	Friday	Saturday	Sunday

Review your week. What was most surprising about this time audit?

_____

_____

_____

Are there items you spent time on you want to eliminate or add?

_____

_____

_____

If you could create your 'perfect' schedule what would it look like?

Monday	Tuesday	Wednesday	Thursday	Friday	Saturday	Sunday

Review your week. How does this 'perfect' week look differently than your current reality?

_____

_____

What is one step you could take to make this schedule your new reality?

_____

How will you feel once you feel in control of your time?

Day 9: More Love, Less Stress

"When the power of love overcomes the power of stress, the world will feel peace." – Jimi Hendrix

Did you know there is an emotion powerful enough to change everything in your life? What if I told you that if you intentionally chose to exude this emotion to yourself and others, everything would change for the better?

The emotion is love. I know it sounds a little strange, but let me explain.

Think about the emotion of love. I want you to picture someone you love so much. How does it feel to be with that person? How do you feel when you think of that person? What would you do for that person? My guess is you feel happy when you are with that person, you feel joy when you think about them, and you would probably do anything for that person.

Love changes everything in your life for the better. Especially when you start with loving the most important person: you.

Loving yourself is transformative. It helps you see the good in yourself and the good in others. It is an emotion so strong it has the power to heal, the power to forgive, the power to overcome.

Now, I want you to think about stress. How does stress feel? Just writing the word made me feel differently. I felt anxious, worried, and upset. I felt out of control. How does stress impact you? Many times, stress negatively impacts all areas of our life. It is a drain on our emotions and actions. I don't know about you, but when I am stressed out about something, it even makes it hard for me to think logically.

These two words—love and stress—affect us in different ways. As you are thinking about what you want more of in your life, my guess is you want more love and less stress. Today, let's reflect on ways you can move closer to having more love and move further away from stress.

Day 9: More Love, Less Stress Questions:

What does stress feel like to you?

_____
_____
_____
_____

What stresses you out the most?

_____
_____
_____
_____

What does love feel like to you?

_____
_____
_____
_____

What fills you with the most love?

_____

_____

_____

_____

Looking at those emotions, do you feel like they are serving the best version of you? Why or why not?

_____

_____

_____

Day 10: More Water, Less Unhealthy Drinks

"Drinking water is like washing out your insides. The water will cleanse the system, fill you up, decrease your caloric load and improve the function of all of your tissues." – Kevin R. Stone

I drink a lot of water and have replaced my sugary drinks and diet sodas with ice tea or water. I try to get at least half my body weight in ounces every day. In my research, I found that many of my problems were coming from not drinking enough water. Did you know if you're dehydrated you'll feel hungry? Or if you're tired, it could be because you need to drink water? Water is so good for you.

For a long time, my husband refused to listen to me about the amount of water he needed to drink. He'd say, "Allison, there's water in my Starbucks coffee." He was right, there is water in coffee, but it doesn't give you the same benefits as drinking plain water.

Lack of water in your body can have many detrimental effects.

After my husband started to drink at least eight eight-ounce bottles of water each day, he was amazed because he felt energized, slept better, didn't feel as worried, his skin looked better, he was able to focus better, and overall he was happier.

Drinking water works; start today!

Here's to a healthier you!

Day 10: More Water, Less Unhealthy Drinks
Questions:

1. How much water do you currently drink in ounces?

_____

2. How many ounces would equal half of your body weight?

_____

3. Now, make a plan to start drinking your water. Do you need a water bottle?

_____

4. If you aren't already a regular water drinker, track your energy level here.

_____

_____

5. Drink your water consistently for one week and re-evaluate how you feel.

_____

_____

Day 11: More Joy, Less Sadness

"Joy is what happens when we allow ourselves to recognize how good things really are." -Marianne Williamson

Have you ever had one of those years when everything seems to go wrong? It seems like nothing is working out how you imagined it should and there's sadness, stress, and hurt in your life.

I think we can all say that at some point, there has been a time in life when it got really difficult. If you are alive, there are going to be changes, challenges, and stressors coming in and out of your life.

So, how do we focus on finding more joy when there is so much negativity?

Joy is defined as a feeling of great pleasure and happiness.

Joy is one of the highest energy emotions you can experience, and if you focus on creating more of it in your life, you'll feel a difference.

If you are focused on sadness, then you'll feel more sadness. There is nothing wrong with being sad or disappointed, but for a long time, I did not understand that I had a choice of choosing my emotions.

What you focus on expands. Do you want to feel more joy? Then focus on it. Do you want to feel sadness? Then focus on it.

Day 11: More Joy, Less Sadness Questions:

Write down the last time something in your life made you sad. Why? What happened? What did you do?

_____

_____

Write down the last time something in your life made you joyful. Why? What happened? What did you do?

_____
_____

Do you enjoy feeling joyful? Why?

_____
_____

What are some actions you can take to feel more joyful in your life?

_____
_____

What are some actions you can take to reduce the sadness in your life?

_____
_____

Reflecting on your answers from above, what is the one thing you could start doing to focus on joy more often?

_____
_____

Day 12: More Happiness, Less Unhappiness

"Who decides whether you shall be happy or unhappy? You do!" – Norman Vincent Peale

That quote changed my life forever. I'm not exaggerating. I never knew I could intentionally create my happiness or unhappiness in life, and so can you.

You can choose today to be happy or not. You have that power within you. Isn't that the best news you've ever heard? Yeah, I think so too.

For the first 20 years of my life, I let everything and everyone else control my happiness. I'd wake up, watch the news, check my social media, and look for negativity in my life. I wasn't aware that I was doing this, but I was not protecting my energy at all.

Did you know that we have access to more information than ever before in history? I saw something that said we receive the same amount of information in one day that some people hundreds of years ago received in their entire lifetimes. WOW, that's kinda crazy.

Are you monitoring the information you are allowing to come to you? Are you filtering information for its impact on your mental and emotional health? I wasn't and I know that this led to me feeling unhappy, worried, and anxious. I hated the feeling, but I did not know what I could do to change it.

Then I read the quote above from Norman Vincent Peale and decided I needed to make some drastic changes.

Here's what I did:

- I quit watching television and news.
- I quit reading online newspapers or blogs.
- I limited my time on social media and blocked negative news.

- I turned off all notifications on my phone and computer (especially news).
- I limited or stopped talking to people who were negative.
- I started to wake up two hours earlier to meditate, pray, read, exercise, and get focused.
- I started to look for the great in every day.
- I started to fill myself up with happy things: people, experiences, music, books, etc.
- I started to read non-fiction books about positive thinking, business, mindset, happiness, emotional intelligence, brain research, human potential, and success principles.
- I found mentorship and a coach to discuss my challenges with.
- I started to create more things to help others: books, podcasts, products, training, etc.
- I put inspirational quotes up everywhere (they are in every room in my house, office, on my phone, etc.).
- I started to exercise, eat healthy foods, and focus on being the healthiest version of myself inside and out.
- I let go of the things that made me sad.

Day 12: More Happiness, Less Unhappiness Questions:

Would you say you are happy or not? Why?

Do you have negative influences that are impacting your happiness? Write them down.

Are there ways you could remove or limit the negative influences from your life?

How would it feel to have more happiness in your life?

What are some actions you can take to increase the happiness in your life?

Reflecting on your answers from today, what is the one thing you could start doing to focus on being happy more often?

What do you need to let go of that makes you sad?

Day 13: More Relaxation, Less Worry

"Our anxiety does not come from thinking about the future, but from wanting to control it." – Kahlil Gibran

I have a friend who was a "worry wort." She worried about everything. Every day she could tell you what to worry about.

I have another friend who is so chill and relaxed I wonder if she ever worries about anything. Every time I see her, she's smiling, relaxed, and exudes overall happiness.

What is the difference between my two friends?

Where they are putting their energy. If you focus on everything that's going wrong in the world or trying to control the future, you can find a lot of things to worry about. However, if you decide to focus on everything that's going right and the things you can control, you'll likely feel more relaxed.

There are so many benefits to relaxation: it helps you reset your brain, calms your nervous system, gives your body physical benefits, heals you, makes you feel happier, makes you feel in control, and helps you get more done (because people like relaxed people).

However, the opposite is also true. Worry can cause you to feel anxious and overwhelmed, not in control, it raises the cortisol levels in your body, put your brain into "flight or fight" mode, and hurts your body.

Just looking at those different options, which one seems like the better option to choose? Relax, friend!

Day 13: More Relaxation, Less Worry

Questions:

What do you worry about most often? Are these things in or out of your control?

_____

_____

Are there ways you could help yourself from spiraling into worrying?

_____

_____

What are some ways you relax?

_____

_____

How would it feel to have more relaxation in your life?

_____

_____

What are some actions you can take to increase the relaxation in your life?

_____

_____

Reflecting on your answers from today, what is the one thing you could start doing to focus on relaxing more often?

_____

_____

Day 14: More Healing, Less Pain

"Healing the world begins with healing yourself." — Grigori Grabovoi

I had a friend recommend an awesome movie on Netflix recently called *Heal*. It shares powerful stories from spiritual leaders, physicians, and those with chronic illnesses that reveal the powerful connection between the human psyche and physical health. The first thing I'd recommend is that you watch this movie if you haven't already.

When you think about healing yourself, you want to consider these areas of your life:

- Physical Health: This is your physical body. If you break your leg, you need to have it fixed. This is the area most people think about when they think about healing their body. This is an important place to start, but there are more things you can do to ensure your overall health and wellness. How are you doing with your physical health?
- Mental/Emotional Health: The thoughts, emotions, and feelings you have internally can have a positive or negative influence on your health. If you are filled with negativity or stress, it can impact your physical and spiritual health. However, if you are filled with positive thoughts and a hopeful attitude, that can make a positive change in your health as well.
- Spiritual Health: If you have a spiritual practice, this can change all areas of life for you. Meditation is a great place to start. Calming your racing thoughts and checking in with your breathing will make a huge difference. Attending religious or spiritual teachings can also make a big difference in your

health and healing.

Your pain or suffering in life can be resolved when you address it. It's okay to ask for help in order to heal. There is no shame in allowing others to see the hurt or pain inside of you. The best thing for you is to heal, and thankfully, there are amazing healers in this world who are committed to helping you heal.

Day 14: More Healing, Less Pain Questions:

Looking at the three areas of health above, which one do you think is most important for you to focus on healing right now?

_____

_____

_____

Do you have any pain in your life right now?

_____

_____

_____

What have you done in the past for your healing?

_____

_____

_____

What's one thing you could do this week to help yourself heal?

_____

_____

Who could help you heal in your mind, body, or spirit? Ideas: Therapist, Coach, Doctor, Naturopath, Personal Trainer, Health Coach, Nutritionist, Massage Therapist, Spiritual Counselor, etc...

_____

_____

Day 15: More Acceptance, Less Judgment

When we shift our thoughts from judging to accepting, not only others but also ourselves, we can restore our happiness."
– Patricia Tashiro

A few years back, I had a friend say something to me in a really critical tone. I automatically judged their behavior and thought, What did I do to deserve to be treated like that?

Each time I thought about the conversation, a whole bunch of judgmental thoughts about her surfaced in my mind. Why would she say that? Did she know it hurt my feelings? What's her deal? I noticed this negative thinking caused me to feel lower energy, exhausted, sad, and upset.

I replayed the conversation over and over in my head and then I realized something profound: Have I ever spoken like that to someone? Have I ever been rude or criticized someone, maybe even unknowingly? Yes, I had. We all have at some point.

The book, A Course in Miracles says, "The ego cannot survive without judgment. The ego seeks to divide and separate. Spirit seeks to unify and heal."

To heal judgment, you need to first become aware of it. The next time you feel yourself judging someone else, take a moment to realize you're doing it and pause. In this pause, recognize the fact that you can choose to let go of the judgment. Don't give it any power. A Course in Miracles: "I choose to judge nothing that occurs."

Choose acceptance. Choose to accept that the other person is doing the best they can today, just like you are. Give yourself a break, and give that other person a break. Choose acceptance today.

Day 15: More Acceptance, Less Judgment

Write down some examples of judgment in your life recently.

_____

_____

_____

Who have you judged and how did it make you feel?

_____

_____

_____

If you were going to take a different perspective on this situation, what could it be?

_____

_____

_____

Practice the pause. What happened?

_____

_____

_____

Once you choose to accept that other person, how did you feel?

_____

_____

_____

Day 16: More Togetherness, Less Separation

"We are more alike, my friends, than we are unalike." – Maya Angelou

In 2018, I flew across the equator to do transformational leadership change in Paraguay with my mentor John Maxwell and a group of coaches. As the airplane landed, I started to realize a big problem. Here I was in a different country with people who spoke a different language, lived in a different way, ate different food, and had different life experiences than me. How would I be able to connect with these people?

Then I arrived in the airport and was greeted by smiles and cheers from a group of excited Paraguayans and I realized how much alike we were. We wanted to love our families, friends, and communities. We wanted to take care of our families' health and wellbeing. We wanted to educate our children and provide access to resources that meet basic needs. We wanted to laugh, smile, and sometimes cry. We wanted justice and we wanted to be accepted.

This trip forever changed me because it helped me realize that deep down, together we are more alike than we are different. When we can see each other as similar and value each other as human, there is a respect and kindness that emerges.

Today, look for a new person to connect with. Ask them questions, get to know them, and be mindful to appreciate your similarities.

This is how we can have more togetherness and less separation.

Day 16: More Togetherness, Less Separation
Questions:

What does the word "together" mean to you and how does it feel?

___

What does the word "separate" mean to you and how does it feel?

___

Have you ever met someone who lives in a different area of the world? What did you have in common?

___

What does togetherness look like in your relationships?

_____

_____

Day 17: More Reading, Less Screen/Computer Time

"The more that you read, the more things you will know. The more that you learn, the more places you'll go." —Dr. Seuss

If there is one thing I could share that would make a HUGE difference in your life, it's this replacement of reading versus screen time. If you've ever spoken to anyone who has reached a high level of success, there's a very good chance that they read books. I'm not talking just about fiction books, but primarily non-fiction books. Reading is magical in the way it allows people to share information. If there's an influential person that you want to learn from, whether they are alive or not, you can probably find a book that they wrote or a book about them. Then you can read about their life. You can learn how they think, how they have created their life, and how they make things happen. This information can help you re-design your life using the information you learned. See, what I mean? Reading is powerful, especially when done in a way that can positively impact your life. I bet you can guess your project for today... go find a book to read and shut off that screen.

Day 17: More Reading, Less Screen/Computer Time Questions:

Open up your phone's screen time tracker to see how many hours per day you are on it. Then do the math. Multiply that number by 365 days. For example, if you are on your phone/

iPad/screen one hour a day x 365 days. That means you spend 365 hours on a screen! Do you think you could replace that time with reading? How could your life look differently if you made that one small change?

Be intentional about your book selection. What are the two to three topics you want to be an expert in? Then choose the bestselling book in those topics to start your reading adventure.

Choose the best time to read. Morning? Lunch? Evening? Late at night?

One important part of reading is gathering what you've learned. How could you track the information you learned in each book? I typically write about the lessons, file, or mind-map the best ideas. What works best for you?

How many books do you want to read this year? Why is this important to your growth?

Day 18: More Nature Time, Less Indoor Time

"Look deep into nature, and then you will understand everything better." — Albert Einstein

Think about the last time you went for a walk outside. What did you experience? Was the sun shining? Wind blowing? How did it smell?

There is something about being outside that allows us to reset. During the spring of 2020 when we were in the shutdown in Wisconsin, I took multiple walks/runs each day in nature. I watched winter turn to spring. Each day I'd notice a small change in nature, from the snow melting into the stream, birds singing, buds on trees, and then into full spring. It was a fun transition to experience and I know that I never could have been so fully present witnessing these changes if I would not have taken the time to be outside in it.

The stream doesn't yell, "Hey, look at this, the snow is melting." The birds don't knock on the door of my house and say, "We're going to be singing this afternoon, come experience it." The trees don't scream, "Watch this, we're creating buds and then one day it'll be leaves… magical." And yet nature does this transformation every day. How often do you take the time to appreciate it? The best part of nature is we can learn from the changes and seasons. Just like there are seasons in nature, there are seasons in life. Just like the streams flow, our lives flow. Birds sing and we have good days. The leaves pop and we experience a change in our lives. Nature and our lives are so similar, but the only way to notice this is to experience it firsthand. Think about the difference between watching a video about a zoo and taking a trip to the zoo to visit the animals. We need to fully experience things in our lives in order to apply them and use them.

Today, I encourage you to go for a walk outside. If it's cold by you, bundle up. If it's hot, bring water. Either way, get outside in nature today.

Day 18: More Nature Time, Less Indoor Time Questions:

Estimate how much time you spend outside right now per day. Why?

_____
_____

Make a plan for how you can spend time outside more frequently.

_____
_____

Create a list of things you'd like to do outside (hobbies/sports).

_____
_____

What do you need to prepare yourself to be outside more often? What shoes/boots, clothing, coats, equipment should you buy to prepare yourself to be outdoors?

_____

How did it feel to go outside? What did you notice?

Day 19: More Intentionality, Less Hustle

"When you intentionally use your everyday life to bring about positive change in the lives of others, you begin to live a life that matters."— John Maxwell

Did you know that hustling may be hurting you? One week I had five podcast interviews and each of the people I interviewed talked about ending the idea that we need to "hustle" in order to be successful. You think that if you just work harder, you'll get to that fictitious place of "success" quicker, but what if that belief is not really true? What if what you've been told is a lie? You see, hustling just for the sake of hustling will ultimately lead to burnout, broken relationships, health issues, financial issues, and a whole bunch of other ugly things.

What is the alternative? Being intentional in your life. Today, you'll be taking time to finally figure out what matters most to you so you can prioritize those things and get rid of the rest. By taking time to truly think about who and what matters the most, you'll be able to spend time on making your life more meaningful and fulfilled. Your life was meant to have alignment, and hustling is not alignment. Alignment comes when you find stillness and balance in your priorities. Alignment comes when you know who you are and when you tap into the power within you on a spiritual level.

Your time is limited. What you decide to prioritize matters. Take the time to get crystal clear about what this means to you and your family. Is work going to be your full focus or your family? Are you going to make a positive contribution in the world using your gifts or are you going to let excuses stop you from pursuing your passions?

My friend, you have this one life... make it the most amazing experience you possibly can.

Day 19: More Intentionality, Less Hustle Questions:

This may seem a bit dark, but I want you to close your eyes and picture your funeral. Someone you love stands up in front of the room and talks about you.

What do they say to describe you and your life?

_____
_____
_____
_____
_____
_____

What were your priorities?

_____
_____
_____

How did you make a difference?

_____
_____
_____
_____

Who and what mattered to you most?

_____
_____
_____

How did you help others using your gifts?

_____
_____
_____

After going through these questions, what do you need to change in your life in order to be in alignment with who you truly are?

_____
_____
_____

Day 20: More Slow, Less Hurry

"Think of life as a marathon." – Clifton Maclin, Jr.

During one conversation with my mentor Clif, he said, "Allison, you are a sprinter in life. You focus on accomplishing something quickly, then take a break. What if you slowed down and thought about life as a marathon?" After he said this, I immediately got defensive. I *am not*, I thought. But now I realize that I was sprinting through my life. I was hurrying through every day. I was so busy I was missing out on the things that truly mattered. We live in a time when life seems to want to go fast, but I'd encourage you to find ways to slllllooooooooooowwwww down.

It's okay to take it easy and give yourself a break. There is a misconception out there that you must "hustle" in order to reach success. Or that you must sacrifice everything in order to become what you truly want to be. I believe this is false. I think that in order to become all that we were meant to be, we really need to slow down and recognize who it is that we want to become.

There were years in my early thirties when I felt lost in who I wanted to become. I sacrificed my relationships, health, and passions for who I thought I "should" be. I wanted approval from people who really did not care what I did, but I thought they did. I was living my life hurried because I was trying to catch who I was. I thought the faster I did the wrong things, the faster I'd figure out what it was I was supposed to do.

Then, after my mentor Cliffy passed away, my heart hurt and I heard his wise words every single day. I heard him remind me to put my faith and my family first. He'd remind me that they are all that truly mattered. I heard him remind me to do things that filled my heart with joy and helped serve others. In honor of Clif,

I started to pour my life into helping others find their passion and their purpose. He told me to believe in myself. This one was the hardest to recognize within me because I was moving so fast. Belief comes in stillness. Belief comes in knowing you are on the path, not necessarily knowing where that path may lead you. As I slowed down, I realized deep down in my soul that I needed to slow down to let belief catch up to me.

It's in the stillness of life that we can get in touch with who we are and what matters. That's when the things that truly matter to your heart have a chance to catch up to you. Remember what you did yesterday? Reflect on what truly matters in your life. In order to make the time for this, you may need to slow your pace a bit. You may have to become more focused and intentional about how you use your time. It's okay to give yourself thinking time or to take a day off. But, by doing this, you'll quickly realize everything you were missing when you were rushing from one thing to another.

Slowing down allows your mind, body, and spirit to recover and reset. This allows you to have more energy when you need it.

Day 20: More Slow, Less Hurry Questions:

Have you been rushing through life? Why?

What's one thing you could do to slow down?

When you are rushing or hurrying, how do your physical body and mind feel?

When you intentionally slow down, how do your physical body and mind feel?

Which of these feelings serves the best version of you more? Why?

Day 21: More Responsibility, Less Blaming Questions

"Everything you do is based on the choices you make. It's not your parents, your past relationships, your job, the economy, the weather, an argument or your age that is to blame. You and only you are responsible for every decision and choice you make. Period." – Dr. Wayne Dyer

This is such a great quote! I have it up in my office to remind myself that I always, always have a choice. Whether or not I like something in my life is completely and totally my responsibility.

Have you thought about the choices that you've made in your life? I know that many times we get caught up in life and never stop to take responsibility for what is happening to us.

As I was going through this reset, I realized I had many areas of life where I was blaming others rather than take full responsibility for my life. I needed to own my life and that included my thoughts, feelings, actions, and behaviors.

Today, I encourage you to be more intentional about whether you are taking full responsibility in your life.

I challenge you to think about the things in your life. Are you taking full responsibility for them?

Day 21: More Responsibility, Less Blaming Questions:

What area of your life have you been making the most

excuses? Spirituality, Family, Friends, Field/Career, Fun, Fitness, Finances

_____

_____

What is one thing you need to start taking responsibility for in your life?

_____

_____

Why is it important to take responsibility for what you wrote down?

_____

_____

_____

Day 22: Which activity was your favorite? Why?

"Sometimes, you have to look back in order to understand the things that lie ahead." — Yvonne Woon

This last week is about reflecting on your journey of resetting your life. This week we'll be mindfully reviewing what you experienced so you can keep the things that helped you and toss the things that did not.

Why are we doing this? Great question. My mentor John Maxwell often says, "Experience isn't the best teacher, evaluated experience is." He encourages his family to evaluate their experiences and take the time to reflect on what they learned and how they grew.

During my life as a wife, parent, sister, business owner, author, etc., I've realized that reflection teaches me so much. Sometimes, I use reflection to learn what went well during a training or event. Other times, I use reflection to remember a conversation or a feeling I experienced. Reflection is an awesome resource that can help us figure out what is working in our life and maybe what is not working and how we want it to work instead.

I'd like you to take some time right now to review what you've experienced over the past 21 days. Take some time to review your notes and think about the activities you felt most connected to. I bet there were a few activities that excited and inspired you. There may have been some activities you didn't like at the time, but a few days later realized the importance it could have in your life.

Reflection will help you evaluate what you like or not. It'll help you recognize what you need more of in your life and what you need less of. It'll help you find focus and calmness. It'll help fill your heart with happiness. Reflection will help you use your own experience to figure out what comes next or what to stop doing. You have many of the answers you are seeking, so take a moment to be calm and reflective. You'll be amazed at what you realize.

Day 22: Which activity was your favorite? Why?

What was your favorite activity? Why?

Day 23: How are you feeling?

"In any given moment, we have two options: to step forward into growth or to step back into safety." — Abraham Maslow

You can tell a lot about where you are in your life by evaluating where you are emotionally. Some people want to deny that they have feelings, but everyone has emotions, and emotions drive our behavior, which leads to the results we get out of life. My guess is that you started this process of resetting your life because you did not feel very good emotionally. Some emotions I felt when I first did my life rest were overwhelmed, anger, frustration, depression, and hopelessness. I was in full burnout and survival zone, and I knew that I needed to do something to reset my life. Perhaps you were not in as extreme place as I was, but you probably were feeling some sort of discomfort.

Here's the thing about emotions: they are clues to how we're doing. If you are feeling negative emotions for many days, you have a clue that something is not healthy inside of you. This emotional awareness can help us to ask for help and get support. There is no shame in asking for help. There is strength and power in saying, "I need help." For too long I suffered in silence. I felt terrible emotionally and it drained my energy and made me feel hopeless.

As soon as I asked for help, I was able to slowly rebuild my emotional wellbeing. Little by little I started to see the good in each day, and eventually, that became a habit. Emotions are clues.

How does your heart feel emotionally? Are you feeling fulfilled and joyful? Do you have great relationships or not? Do you feel like the healthiest version of yourself? Are you able to do the things you want to do to help the people you love helping?

Your emotional health will impact every single area of your life. If you are depressed, anxious, or hopeless, it's time to find help processing those emotions. There is strength and courage gained in finding help for yourself. The best part is, as soon as you seek out help, you'll start to feel lighter and better.

My hope is that after 22 days of intentionally centering your mind, body, and spirit, you feel pretty great, but there is a chance that you may need more help. Please look for it. It may be a therapist, a doctor, or a friend. It's 100% okay and 100% helpful to ask for help. Your mental health will impact every other area of your life, so making sure you have support to be the healthiest version of yourself is important.

Day 23: How are you feeling?

Reflect on your emotions when you started the Reset Your Life process.

_____

_____

Now, how are you feeling today emotionally?

_____

_____

What do you think shifted in you to make the change in your emotions?

_____

Day 24: What's one fun thing you could do today? Do it!

"There's not a shred of evidence that life is serious." – funny card

When I was in college, I received a card from a friend that said, "There's not a shred of evidence that life is serious." It had a funny-looking dog in a car. I remember laughing out loud, and this was after weeks of feeling lonely.

Friends, I'm going to tell you a very big secret. YOU CAN HAVE FUN!

Your life can be a fun adventure. You can laugh. You can make surprises happen. You can dance, play, and decorate things for no good reason! Yes, people may think you are crazy, but while you're enjoying life, those people can say whatever the heck they want because you'll be having fun.

When I was a non-profit leader, I was charged with growing a board in the middle of nowhere in a snowstorm. I am not kidding. I remember trying to figure out how in the world I was going to convince people to drive and one to two hours to our meetings each month in a white-out snowstorm in the middle of nowhere.

Then one day, I figured out the solution. I'd make it fun. I decorated the room, brought in toys, candy, played games, had tropical parties in winter, pizza parties, played loud music, gave out awards, blew up balloons, and one time I stopped traffic by having a clown lead a parade down the main street. (That one got us on the front page of the newspaper! Oh, and the cops and firefighters came… I invited them.) We had fun and we made positive change happen in early childhood.

Fun brings success! Seriously, have more fun. Even if you are an adult, you are able to have fun, laugh, and enjoy your life. I know it may seem crazy, but it's true. And the people in your life will enjoy the fact that you are intentionally creating fun experiences too. There's a positive ripple effect when you are having fun.

My point is that for some reason when you become a teenager or adult, you think you can't have fun anymore. That's crap! You can have fun; life was meant to be enjoyed.

Day 24: What's one fun thing you could do today? Do it!

Write a list of fun things you want to do but have been putting off. Now circle one and do it... TODAY!

_____

_____

_____

_____

_____

_____

_____

_____

Day 25: Celebrate your accomplishments, write them down.

"What you focus on grows, what you think about expands, and what you dwell upon determines your destiny." — Robin S. Sharma

Did you know that we all are built with a negativity bias? This essentially means if we are not aware of it, we think negatively about ourselves about 70% of the time. YUCK! So, here's the deal: in order to rewrite that negativity, you need something positive to fill your brain with. It needs to be powerful and true about who you are or who you want to become.

Today your job is to honor your awesomeness. YES, YOU! No, you are not "bragging" by writing down your accomplishments; you are honoring your greatness. You are honoring your strengths, talents, and accomplishments. This is an important and critical step to rewriting those negative beliefs about yourself that come so easily.

Here's the truth: what you tell your brain about you it believes. If you call yourself a cotton-headed ninny muggins (like Elf), your brain will believe that you are a cotton-headed ninny muggins. Get it?

Now, if you fill your brain with your accomplishments and positive attributes, your brain will believe them too. I know what you're thinking right now: "Allison you're brilliant, let me pay you one bazillion dollars for your brilliance because this stuff is going to seriously transform my entire life!!!!!" Yes, I know!

Right now, I want you to close your eyes, take a deep breath, and center yourself. Picture yourself as the best version of yourself.

Think about your life and when you have felt the best about yourself. What were you doing? Who were you with? How did it feel? If you are thinking that you have never felt that way, then you need to think harder, because I believe that everyone has had a time in their life when they felt the most alive.

Day 25: Celebrate your accomplishments, write them down

Right now, write down all of your accomplishments! EVERYTHING! (If you need help ask a loved one or friend for ideas of awesome things you've done. Get more paper if needed.)

_____

_____

_____

_____

_____

_____

_____

_____

_____

_____

Day 26: Create a list of 10 positive words to describe yourself. Read them out loud daily.

"Just believe in yourself. Even if you don't, pretend that you do and at some point you will." – Venus Williams

My daughter is five years old right now, and if you ask her what I do, she says, "My mama is a believer in people." I didn't think of my job like that until she continued to ask me if I was going to "believe in people again."

I do believe in you. I think it's exciting to believe in people and see their potential. I've heard that only 2% of people ever reach their full potential. That's means we have about 98% of the population that is missing a key ingredient of success: BELIEF.

Belief in yourself is the first step to everything. Unfortunately, as I've spoken to more and more people from all over the world, I hear doubt and fear dominating many people's thoughts. This is especially present when someone is growing themselves in some area of life. Growth is difficult and it actually entails you becoming a different version of yourself. For most of us, when we start to transform our lives in some area, say our health, it means we need to replace our old bad habits with new healthy habits that align with the vision of our best self. Here's the trick: the other thing that must change is your beliefs. If you continue to tell yourself that you are unhealthy and eat unhealthly, there is NO way you will ever reach your goal of being healthy. It's not possible because you are reaffirming to yourself exactly the opposite of what you want to have happened.

Instead, you need to consciously affirm what it is you need to have happened. For example, when I decided to get healthier in my own life, I had to switch the belief that I hated working out. I knew that would not serve the healthiest version of myself, and so I switched that belief to "I love working out, it makes me feel strong and confident." At first saying, this felt like a lie, but eventually, my brain realized I was not kidding and now I really do love working out and it truly does make me feel strong and confident.

You are what you believe. If you believe you are worthy, amazing, and wonderful... then you are.

Talking to yourself with kindness and love can shift everything in your life. It'll make bad days good. It'll repair broken relationships with forgiveness. It'll give you strength and courage, even when you're afraid. It'll give you energy and excitement, even when you are tired. Powerful words will change everything if you let them.

Today that changes because you are the boss of you.

Day 26: Create a list of 10 positive words to describe yourself. Read them out loud daily.

Visualization Activity:

- *Please, close your eyes.*

- *Imagine your best day ever.*

What are you doing?

_____

_____

_____

Who is with you?

_____

_____

_____

How does it feel?

_____

_____

_____

Where are you?

_____

_____

_____

Now, write down words to describe the most powerful best version of yourself.

_____

_____

Day 26: Create a list of 10 positive words to describe yourself. Read them out loud daily.

Day 27: Thank yourself for being committed to growth.

"Gratitude opens the door to ... the power, the wisdom, the creativity of the universe." – Deepak Chopra

You're almost finished with your *Reset Your Life* process. This has been a journey of growth for you and now is the time to thank yourself for taking time for your personal development. You are important, and by carving out the time to do this, you've proven to yourself that you can make important things happen in your life.

Being thankful for the journey is the key to reaching any destination. You have committed to your own growth and that is something awesome to celebrate.

When I was starting my own personal development journey, I had a mentor tell me, "Allison, start to celebrate more." I thought this sounded ridiculous. I politely asked, "Why?"

"Allison, in order to get more of that thing into your life, you must celebrate what you want more of."

I felt like someone shared the most powerful secret with me. Put energy into what I want more of in my life. Up to that point, I had been spending way too much time putting energy into the exact opposite of what I wanted in my life. Have you ever had a bad day and then went around telling everyone why it was so horrible? Now think about how many times you had a fantastic day and celebrated it (birthdays don't count). If you're anything like me, you probably haven't ever done it.

Today I want you to be thankful and celebrate this journey you've gone through. You've taken the time and energy to become a different version of yourself. You're probably feeling different about yourself and are more excited about your future. Your heart may feel full and grateful. This is exactly the right time to celebrate!

Being thankful and showing gratitude in your life is a great practice. By simply writing down a few things you are grateful for each day, you train your mind and heart to search for the good in life.

Day 27: Thank yourself for being committed to growth.

Write yourself a thank you letter. Congratulate yourself for your commitment, strength, and growth. Let yourself know how this will change who you are from now on.

_____
_____
_____
_____
_____
_____
_____
_____
_____
_____
_____
_____
_____

Day 28: More Abundance, Less Scarcity

"If you look at what you have in your life, you'll always have more. If you look at what you don't have in life, you'll never have enough." - Oprah Winfrey

Abundance is an amazing tool. Abundance means that if you have one pie, there are unlimited pieces for others. Scarcity says if you have a pie, you have limited pieces so you better protect your pie and not share it with others.

Abundance means more.

Scarcity means less.

In life, abundance means you have the mindset that you have more than enough, and as a result, you'll start to feel the infinite power of the universe conspiring for your highest good. Life will start to work out in your favor. Things may not be perfect, but you'll start to appreciate life in a new way and you'll start to serve others in a bigger way.

Scarcity keeps you stuck in the mindset that you are in competition with, well, everyone. You think you're in some sort of race to nowhere and there is nothing that can fulfill the need to do more, be more, and have more. You'll likely feel drained, lost, and yearning for more when you are in scarcity mode. You'll compare your life, your possessions, your "luck," your career/business, your weight, and anything else to what others have and think... well, I wish I was that lucky.

When you grasp the power of abundance, you'll start to see the fact that there is more than enough, so why can't you take responsibility for your life and go after it? Why not? Because there is more than enough!

Day 28: More Abundance, Less Scarcity
Questions:

If you were going to evaluate your mindset as more abundant or more scarcity-focused, what would you say it is? Why?

_____

_____

_____

What is something in your life you could see as abundant?

_____

_____

_____

What is something in your life you have seen as scarce?

_____

_____

_____

How will focusing on the abundance in your life shift your mindset?

_____

_____

Day 29: Pay it forward!

Definition of Pay it Forward: Pay it forward is an expression for when the recipient of an act of kindness does something kind for someone else rather than simply accepting or repaying the original good deed.

You did it!! YAY for you. You've *Reset Your Life*. How are you feeling? My hope is that you feel more focused, lighter, happier, and ready to tackle life with an abundance mindset. I wish you a life of positivity, fun, laughter, love, hope, and kindness.

Now, this is the final project and it may be the most important step. You'll take what you learned and you'll pay it forward. Paying it forward means that you'll share it with someone in your life who you think this book may help. The person may be your significant other, child, friend, co-worker, client, customer, barista, teacher, or someone you sit next to at your favorite café.

You need to tell them about *Reset Your Life* because it might be the answer they've been praying and hoping for. You never know who in your life is struggling in silence. They are praying for a way to live their life happier, but don't know where to start. There is a yearning in their heart to following their purpose, but they are allowing distractions to stop them.

When you share this book, let the person know how it's positively impacted you. What is one thing you realized about yourself that you really like? What has changed in your thinking? How has it helped you repair relationships (even with yourself)? How has it impacted your health and wellbeing?

Your story will inspire others; share it with more people.

Pay it forward!

Day 29: Pay it forward!

Write down a list of people you want to share Reset Your Life with?

_____
_____
_____

How has this process reset your life?

_____
_____
_____
_____
_____
_____
_____
_____

Day 30: Review of Your Reset

Over the past 30 days, you have reset so many areas of your life.

- You've become more intentional in your life.
- You've spoken to yourself with love, kindness, and positive words.
- You've taken care of your physical body with nutritious food and water.
- You've also moved your body to break a sweat.
- You've stepped out into nature and experienced the calming effect nature has on you.
- You've quit some things that have been filling your life with busyness, but not the impact you needed to be fulfilled.
- You've shifted your emotions.
- You've evaluated your self-talk.
- You've practiced gratitude by either writing down what you are grateful for or acting out gratefulness by sharing something with others.
- You've grown in your awareness of what fills your heart with happiness and love and what does not.
- You've learned that being intentional is better than hustling.
- You've connected with the people in your life.
- You've even connected with yourself in a deep and meaningful way.
- You've sat in silence, listening and observing your thoughts, without judgment.
- You've meditated.
- You've walked.
- You've laughed, had fun, and celebrated.
- You've reflected.
- In this process, you've grown, intentionally.
- You've grown in your mind, body, and spirit.
- You've become someone different than you were 30 days ago.

- You've transformed.

Day 30: Review of Your Reset Questions:

What is the date today?

_____

What was the date 30 days ago?

_____

What happened when you took a social media break?

_____

Right now, how would you rate your current stress/ overwhelm level 1-10 (10 being really stressed out)?

_____

How do you feel now, after going through the reset? Go back to Day 1 to review how you wanted to feel at the end of the month.

_____

If you were going to describe the emotions you feel most during the day now, what would you say they are?

Looking at those emotions, do you feel like they are serving the best version of you? Why or why not?

Thank You

First off, thank you to my husband, best friend, and business partner, Tony Liddle. Your love, encouragement, and kindness touch my heart every day. I love you!

My kids, Avery and Logan teach me so much about life each day. They have helped me realize how important it is to honor your giftedness and just be you. I'm so proud of you two. You two amaze me each day and I'm so grateful God chose me to be your Mama. Love you!

My sister, Anika, and brother, Reid are two of my favorite people on the planet. They are intelligent and brilliant in so many ways. Thank you for being awesome.

During one of the hardest times in my life, my cousin Heidi Stender was my support person. She was always available for a call, text, and ideas. She encouraged me to take care of myself when I needed the reminder. Thank you Heidi for helping me *Reset My Life*, so I could help others learn how to do the same. Love ya!

I thank all of my GREAT family for being loving, kind, and teaching me so many life lessons. I'm grateful to all of you. If I listed all of you it would be an entire book. You know who you are, and I love you immensely.

I thank all my AMAZING mentors and friends for teaching me so much and coming into my life at just the right time. I owe you each my gratitude for your willingness to pour into me with your wisdom and support.

I thank my editor, Danielle Anderson, for her keen eye (again x 4 books!). I seriously could not write these books without your help.

To my readers, I thank all of you for reading this book and supporting my CRAZY huge goals. The best gift is hearing how you moved forward in your life from the words you read in this book. I believe in you. Let me know your success stories at www.allisonliddle.com. God bless!

About the Author

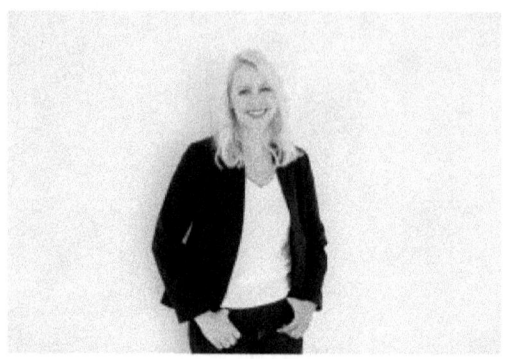

Allison Liddle is a best-selling author of *Life Under Construction: Designing a Life You Love*, *The Art of Imperfect Action: All Success Comes From Daring to Begin and Keep Going: How to Create a Champion Mindset*. *Reset Your Life in 30 Days: A Detox For You Mind, Body & Spirit* is her fourth book.

Allison is a top motivational speaker, leadership trainer, podcast host, CEO/Founder of Allison Liddle Consulting, President of Prosper Wealth Management, and mother to two. Allison's companies have won national industry awards and trained leaders in the Top 10 of the Fortune 500. Allison is passionate about helping high achievers launch to the next level in their lives personally and professionally.

With a winning style that includes a vibrant, upbeat personality combined with her knowledge of proven business-building techniques, Allison is the expert who will help lead you to success. Allison Liddle is an experienced keynote speaker, corporate trainer, and executive coach who brings energy, enthusiasm, and motivation to audiences large and small. Allison connects with each person in the room through her personal stories and life experiences.

Her company, Allison Liddle Consulting helps high achievers launch to the next level in their lives. They do this by creating media, products, events, inspiration, and a tribe that equips them with the leadership and personal growth tools to get the results they want in their lives. They are passionate about helping people reach their goals and build profitable businesses.

Connect with her at allisonliddle.com.

Life Under Construction: Designing a Life You Love
By Allison Liddle

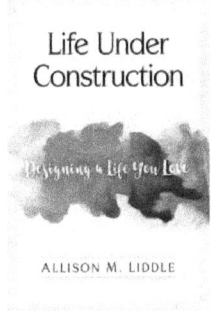

Have you ever felt like your life was under construction? Do you feel stuck in a life that you didn't choose?

Maybe you're starting a new business or career, getting married, having children, retiring, or moving to a new place? Are you trying to get healthier? Or maybe you decided that enough was enough and started to grow yourself into a better version of yourself.

Whatever your life under construction story is, you need help and support. You need to know there are other people that are designing a life that they love too.

In her book, Allison shares her story of when her life was under construction literally. She built a house, an office, had a baby, rebranded a business, and was on a mission to grow herself personally and professionally. The change of designing a life you love can be stressful at times. Change can be hard. Some days you may want to give up and just eat cookies. Allison has been through it all and through her journey has learned some important lessons she would like to share with you.

This book is available on Amazon.

The Art of Imperfect Action: All Success Comes From Daring to Begin

By Allison Liddle

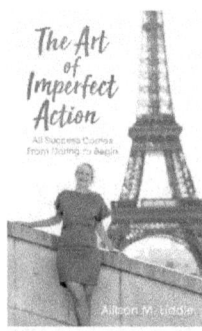

Trust that you are the person to do that thing you're afraid of doing.

Do you have big goals–but haven't taken action on them? Do you wish you could do more, but feel stuck? Do you have the best ideas, but never use them?

Imperfect Action: the act of letting go of perfectionism to take bold, courageous action. Bravery requires you taking the first step toward your goals. Be brave. You have an opportunity right now to step into your greatness. Through this book, you'll get the practical tools you need to move forward in your life. You'll understand some of the reasons you may feel stuck and how to break through them. You'll be equipped, energized, and ready to create massive success in your life through practicing the art of imperfect action! Remember: Commit to your dreams, be courageous, and take imperfect action!

This book is available on Amazon.

Keep Going: How to Create a Champion Mindset

By Allison Liddle

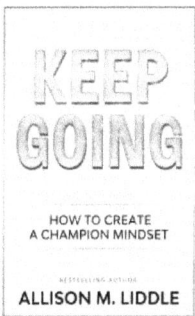

"Consistent champions think and act very differently than non-champions. It is a mindset, a hardwired way of thinking and doing." -Clifton Maclin

Have you ever wondered what makes some people achieve more than others? What do champions who have reached the pinnacle of success do that's different? In "KEEP GOING: How to Create a Champion Mindset," Allison Liddle shares the lessons she learned from her mentors for having the champion mindset daily. You too can learn the powerful lessons of how to keep going and how to create the mindset of a champion. The steps will transform your life, your leadership, and your business to 'KEEP GOING.'

NOTES:

www.ingramcontent.com/pod-product-compliance
Lightning Source LLC
Chambersburg PA
CBHW070302100426
42743CB00011B/2316